YOUR KNOWLEDGE HAS VALUE

- We will publish your bachelor's and
  master's thesis, essays and papers

- Your own eBook and book -
  sold worldwide in all relevant shops

- Earn money with each sale

Upload your text at www.GRIN.com
and publish for free

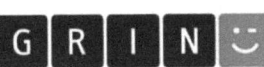

Formulation, Development and Textural Characterization of Nano-Engineering Strategy Assisted Topical Antifungal Nanolipogel

Unnati Patel

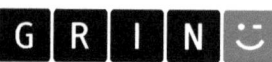

Bibliographic information published by the German National Library:

The German National Library lists this publication in the National Bibliography; detailed bibliographic data are available on the Internet at http://dnb.dnb.de.

ISBN: 9783346972132
This book is also available as an ebook.

© GRIN Publishing GmbH
Trappentreustraße 1
80339 München

Print and binding: Books on Demand GmbH, Norderstedt, Germany
Printed on acid-free paper from responsible sources.

The present work has been carefully prepared. Nevertheless, authors and publishers do not incur liability for the correctness of information, notes, links and advice as well as any printing errors.

GRIN web shop: https://www.grin.com/document/1417665

FORMULATION, DEVELOPMENT AND TEXTURAL CHARACTERIZATION OF NANO-ENGINEERING STRATEGY ASSISTED TOPICAL ANTIFUNGAL NANOLIPOGEL

Patel Unnati[a]

[a]Department of Quality Assurance (PG), Sanjivani College of Pharmaceutical Education and Research, Kopargaon, Maharashtra-423603, India.

Abstract

The aim of the present research work was to formulate, develop and characterize topical antifungal nanolipogel using hundred-times-washed cow ghee base known as *shatadhautaghrita*. It is used as a permeation enhancer to increase the permeation rate of fluconazole. Nine formulations of nanolipogel were prepared using different concentrations of carbopol and *shatadhautaghrita*. The optimized batch of nanolipogel (formulation F7) was evaluated for pH, percentage yield, drug content, extrudability, rheology. The consistency, spreadability and formation of nanosize particles were assessed through texture profile analysis and zetasizer. *In-vitro* drug release and *ex-vivo* permeation studies were performed using Franz diffusion cell apparatus and showen highest values of F7 (80.50% and 83.65%), when compared with commercial gel (0.5%). The highest antifungal activity was seen by using *Candida albicans*was as a model fungus.From the present study, it is concluded that nanolipogel is better formulation for increasing the release, permeation rate and antifungal activity of topical preparation.

Keywords: Topical nanolipogel,*shatadhautaghrita*, fluconazole, permeation, particle size.

Introduction

Fluconazole (FLZ) is an antifungal agent used mainly in topical formulations to treat various skin disorders such as oropharyngeal candidiasis, cryptoccocal meningitis and cutaneous dermatophyte infections. FLZ is a synthetic triazole derivative that acts as an antifungal. FLZ preferentially inhibits fungal cytochrome P-450 sterol C-14 alpha-demethylation[5].

Shatadhautaghrita(SDG)isused as a natural permeation enhancer in topical products[20]. It is prepared by washing cow ghee 100 times with water.*shatadhautaghrita* is (*shata* = one hundred, *dhauta* = washed) clarified butter fat that has been washed 100 times[18]. The use of *shatadhautaghrita* in managing conditions such as burns, chicken pox, scars, wounds, herpes, leprosy and other skin diseases and as a vehicle for drugs for external application are mentioned in traditional texts. The characteristic odour and granular, oily consistency of cow ghee are not present in *shatadhautaghrita*, and so it is a homogeneous, smooth, non-oily product that is easier to apply. The neutral pH of *shatadhautaghrita* compared with the acidic pH value of ghee makes *shatadhautaghrita* beneficial by preventing skin irritation. The reduced particle size of *shatadhautaghrita* makes the product non-granular, non-sticky and homogeneous, which makes it easy to apply it on the skin and may result in an increased rate of absorption through the skin. Washing results in a homogeneous oil-in-water emulsion with better consistency and viscosity, which makes it suitable for use in topical applications[3, 13].

FLZ is a Class III drug having low permeability and high solubility. Hence it is necessary to increase its permeability so that the desired bioavailability is achieved[19]. This is needed for formulating topical dosages. The aim of the present study was to prepare a topical antifungal nanolipogel (NLG) using the hundred-times-washed cow ghee base known as *shatadhautaghrita*. It may be used as a permeation enhancer to increase the permeation rate of fluconazole.

3

Materials And Methods

Fluconazole was received as a gift from Cipla Pharmaceuticals Ltd., Mumbai. Carbopol 934P, propylene glycol, triethanolamine, propylparaben and methylparaben were of pharmaceutical grade and obtained from Research Lab Fine Chem Industries, Mumbai. The solvents used were of analytical grade.

Methods

Preparation of ShataDhautaGhrita

Copper vessels were used to prepare *shatadhautaghrita*. The vessels were cleaned thoroughly and rinsed with purified water. 2.5 kg cow ghee was taken in one copper vessel, and 1.5 L of purified water was added to it. The mixture of cow ghee and water was mixed for 15–20 minutes in a Kenwood apparatus. The contents of the vessel were allowed to settle down. The water was decanted carefully, avoiding any loss of ghee. A fresh slot of 1.5 L purified water and previously washed cow ghee was taken, and the same procedure was repeated. This operation was carried out 100 times to obtain *shatadhautaghrita*. Sample of the *shatadhautaghrita* was collected and stored in copper containers at room temperature.[3].

Preparation of Nanolipogel

Carbopol 934P and purified water were taken in a beaker, and the Carbopol 934P was allowed to soak for 24 hours. Fluconazole was dissolved in propylene glycol and added to the above solution. Other excipients (methylparaben and propylparaben) were also added. The pH value of the gels was brought to skin pH using triethanolamine. The final weight of the gel was adjusted to 100 g with purified water. After this gel base was prepared, the *shatadhautaghrita* was added with continuous stirring. Nine nanolipogel formulations were prepared using different concentrations of Carbopol and *shatadhautaghrita*. These formulations were evaluated on the basis of physical stability and phase separation. Table I below provides the compositions of the nine formulations[14, 16].

This article does not contain any studies with human or animal subjects as it performed by any of the authors for in-vivo study, but the Ex-vivo study contains the goat abdominal skin. So all institutional and national guidelines for the care and use of laboratory animals were followed

Table I. Composition of formulation batches(100g) (% w/w)

Ingredients (%)	F1	F2	F3	F4	F5	F6	F7	F8	F9
Fluconazole	0.5	0.5	0.5	0.5	0.5	0.5	0.5	0.5	0.5
SDG	30	50	70	30	50	70	30	50	70
Carbopol-934P	0.35	0.25	0.15	0.7	0.5	0.3	1.05	0.75	0.45
Propylene Glycol	5.95	4.25	2.55	5.95	4.25	2.55	5.95	4.25	2.55
Methyl Paraben	0.007	0.005	0.003	0.007	0.005	0.003	0.007	0.005	0.003
Propyl Paraben	0.035	0.025	0.015	0.035	0.025	0.015	0.035	0.025	0.015
Triethanolamine	1.05	0.75	0.45	1.05	0.75	0.45	1.05	0.75	0.45
Purified Water	62	44	26	62	50	26	61	43	26

SDG, *shata dhauta ghrita.*

Characterization of *ShataDhautaGhrita* and Nanolipogel

Drug–excipients compatibility studies

Differential scanning calorimetry (DSC)

DSC studies were performed on the drug, the physical mixtures and a 1:1 drug–carbopol mixture. The samples (3–4 mg) were placed on an aluminium pan and heated at a rate of 0°C/minute to a temperature of 200°C using a differential scanning calorimeter (Metler Toledo)[5].

Fourier transform infrared spectrophotometry (FTIR)

FTIR studies were carried out on the drug using an FTIR spectrophotometer (FT-IR 8400; Shimadzu Co., Kyoto, Japan) and the formation of nanolipogel was determined using an FTIR spectrophotometer (JASCO-4600LE) with an ATR Pro ONE accessory. The disks were scanned over the wave number range 4000–400 cm^{-1})[5].

Physical examination

The *shatadhautaghrita* and nanolipogel formulation were inspected visually for colour, homogeneity, consistency and spreadability[11].

pH determination

The pH values of the *shatadhautaghrita* and nanolipogel were determined using a digital pH meter (PICO+ pH meter, LAB INDIA). One gram of each sample was added to 100 ml of distilled water and stored for 2 hours. The pH values of the *shatadhautaghrita* and nanolipogel were determined in triplicate, and the average values were calculated[15].

Percentage yield

An empty container was weighed. The gel formulation was transferred to it, and the container was weighed with the gel formulation. The weight of the empty container was subtracted from the weight of the container with the gel formulation, giving the practical yield. Then the percentage yield was calculated using the formula[2]

$$\text{Percentage yield} = \frac{\text{Practical yield}}{\text{Theoretical yield}} \times 100$$

Drug content

The drug content was determined by dissolving 1 g of the formulation in phosphate buffer of pH 6.8. The solution was stirred continuously for 2 hours using a magnetic stirrer. The resultant solution was transferred to a 100 ml flask, and the final volume adjusted to 100 ml using phosphate buffer of pH 6.8. After suitable dilution of the drug, the absorbance was determined using a UV–visible spectrophotometer at 258 nm with a phosphate buffer of pH 6.8[8].

Tube extrudability

A collapsible aluminium tube was filled with the gel formulation. The tube was pressed to extrude the material, and the extrudability of the formulation was checked[4]. Shown in Table III.

Rheological study

Rheology may be defined as the science concerned with the deformation of matter under increased stress, which may be applied perpendicular to the surface of a body, tangential to the surface of the body or at any angle to the surface of the body.

Rheological studies were carried out on the optimized batch of the nanolipogel formulation using a Brookfield viscometer (RST-CC Rheometer) with coaxial cylinder spindles using the following four blocks:

(1) Rotation ramp measuring block. CSS. lin. 0 -> 50 Pa 60 s. M points

(2) Rotation ramp measuring block. CSS. lin. previous value -> 0 Pa 60 s. 6 M points

(3) Analysis basics

(4) Thixotropy.

Non-Newtonian systems such as plastics, pseudoplastics and dilatant systems show time-dependent changes in the viscosity at varying shearing stresses at a given temperature. This behaviour is known as thixotropy[16, 1].

Texture profile analysis

Texture profile analysis (TPA) of the *shatadhautaghrita* and nanolipogel (F7) was performed using a CT3 texture analyser in TPA mode. The formulations were transferred into the lower cone. Care was taken to avoid introducing air into the samples. A conical analytical probe (45°) was forced down into each sample at a defined test speed (2 mm/second) and to a defined depth (12 mm). At least five replicate analyses of each sample were performed at 25°C and at 30°C. From the resulting force–time plots, the hardness (the force required to attain a given deformation), compressibility (the work required to deform the product during the first pass of the probe) and adhesiveness (the work necessary to overcome the attractive forces between the surface of the sample and the surface of the probe) were derived[10,6].

Spreadability test

Spreadability denotes the area over which a topical formulation spreads when applied to affected parts of the skin. A spreadability test was carried out on the *shatadhautaghrita* and nanolipogel (F7) using a CT3 texture analyser in compression mode. The formulations were transferred into the lower cone. Care was taken to avoid introducing air into the samples. A conical analytical probe (45°) was forced down into each sample at a defined test speed (2 mm/second) to a defined depth (12 mm). At least five replicate analyses of each sample were performed at temperatures of 25°C and 30°C. From the resulting force–time plots, the firmness and the spreadability were derived[17].

Particle size

The particle sizes of the *shatadhautaghrita* and nanolipogel (F7) were measured using a Malvern zetasizer (Ver. 6.20). The mean particle size and particle size distribution (PDI) were determined using this equipment.

In-vitro drug release study

An *in-vitro* drug release study of the gel was performed using a cellophane dialysis membrane and modified Franz diffusion cell apparatus. The cellophane membrane was soaked in phosphate buffer (pH 6.8) for 24 hours. The membrane was cut into circles of diameter 3 cm. The receptor compartment was filled with phosphate buffer (pH 6.8). The temperature was maintained at 37±0.5°C using a water jacket. 0.5 gm of the nanolipogel was uniformly spread on the cellophane membrane. The solution in the receptor compartment of the Franz diffusion cell was continuously stirred at 50 rpm using a magnetic stirrer. At specific time intervals, 1 ml of the solution was taken out and immediately replaced with 1 ml of fresh phosphate buffer solution. The concentration of the drug was determining using UV spectrophotometry at 258 nm[12].

Ex-vivo drug permeation study

A percutaneous permeation study of the gel was carried out using modified Franz diffusion cell apparatus. The membrane used was goat abdominal skin. The skin was cut into circles of diameter 3 cm. Prepared skin samples (goat skin) were mounted on the receptor compartment of the permeation cell with the stratum corneum facing upward and the dermis side facing downward. The donor compartment was kept on the receptor compartment and secured tightly with clamps. The receptor compartment was then filled with 10 ml of pH 6.8 phosphate buffer. The temperature of the medium was maintained at 37±0.5°C using a temperature-controlled water jacket. 0.5 gm of the nanolipogel was spread uniformly on the skin. The solution in the receptor compartment of the Franz diffusion cell was continuously stirred at 50 rpm with a magnetic stirrer. At specific time intervals, 1 ml of the solution was taken out and immediately replaced with 1 ml of fresh phosphate buffer solution. The concentration of the drug was determining by UV spectrophotometry at 258 nm[10].

Antifungal activity study

Fluconazole acts as a fungistatic and inhibits the biosynthesis of ergosterol, the major sterol found in the fungal cell membrane. The prepared formulation was tested using agar well diffusion against *Candida albicans* stain. Sabouraud dextrose agar was prepared, and the fungal stain (*Candida albicans*) was dispersed in the medium. The medium was poured into a sterile Petri plate and allowed to cool to room temperature. Once it solidified, 6 mm wells were cut using a flamed cork borer. Each of the wells was filled with the prepared formulation and a commercial formulation (0.5%) using a sterile syringe. Each well was observed and the diameter of inhibition calculated and compared with that of the commercial formulation [9, 7].

10

Results

Nine nanolipogel formulations were prepared using different concentrations of Carbopol 934P and *shatadhautaghrita*. Batch F7 was selected for further evaluation on the basis of physical stability. Other batches showed phase separation or instability.

Drug–excipient compatibility studies

Any formulation development work has to be preceded by preformulation studies. This preformulation study includes drug-excipients compatibility deliberate by DSC and FT-IR analysis.

DSC

The DSC thermogram of fluconazole is characterized by one sharp endothermic peak at about 139°c, which corresponds to the melting point of fluconazole. The DSC scan of physical mixture also showed a sharp melting at 139°C. It is clear that there is no change in the position of the characteristic peak of the drug in the physical mixture with carbopol. The gel formulation showed a melting point at 124°C indicates slight alteration of melting point it was assumed that the interaction of *shatadhautaghrita* responsible for alteration of melting point.. This indicates there was no interaction between the drug and all the polymers used in the preparation of gel. The results are shown in Figure 1.

FTIR

The FTIR study showed that there was no major change in the position of the peak obtained in the nanolipogel formulation compared with the drug. This shows that there was no interaction between the drug and the excipients even with the SDG. The results are shown in Figure 2 (a) and (b) and Figure 8 .

Physical examination

The *shatadhautaghrita* and nanolipogel formulations were white and viscous, with a smooth, consistent and homogeneous appearance. They were easily spreadable and considered acceptable patients compliance to avoid the risk of irritation upon application to the skin. Shown in Table II.

Table II. Appearance and pH of *shata dhauta ghrita* and nanolipogel

Sr. No.	Formulation	Appearance	pH
1	SDG	White, Smooth, Non oily	6.1±0.27
2	NLG (F7)	White, Smooth, Viscous	7.2±0.15

SDG, *shata dhauta ghrita*; NLG, nanolipogel.

Percentage Yeild

The percentage yield of optimized formulation was found to be 98.45%.

Table III: Percentage yield,drug content (%) and tube extrudability of nanolipogel

Percentage Yield(%)	Drug Content (%)	Tube Extrudability
98.45	97.12±0.19	Excellent

Rheological study

Rheological studies were performed on a Brookfield viscometer (RST-CC rheometer) with coaxial cylinder spindles. The shear stress, shear rate and viscosity data generated for the optimized nanolipogel batch (F7) was used to understand the characteristics of the nanolipogel. The results of the rheological studies indicate that the formulation was a non-Newtonian system (dilatant) because the viscosity of the nanolipogel changes with a change in the applied shear force.

The results of the thixotropy analysis indicate that the formulation was a non-Newtonian system (dilatant) because as the shear rate changed the formulation showed a change in viscosity. All the rheograms and the results of thixotropy analysis are shown in Figures 3(a) and (b), respectively. The shear stress, shear rate, viscosity and temperature data are shown in Table IV.

Table IV : Data of rheological study

Sr. No.	Time (s)	Shear Stress	Shear Rate (1/s)	Viscosity (Pa.s)	Temp (ºC)
	T	(Pa) τ	γ	η	T
1	10	0.000	0.000	0.0000	1000.0
2	20	9.984	0.000	0.0000	1000.0
3	30	19.989	0.022	906.6497	1000.0
4	40	29.993	0.065	462.5318	1000.0
5	50	39.998	0.185	215.6723	1000.0
6	60	49.982	0.654	76.4675	1000.0
1	70	49.998	0.888	56.2622	1000.0
2	80	39.998	0.441	90.7092	1000.0
3	90	29.993	0.195	154.1773	1000.0
	100	19.989	0.039	513.7682	1000.0
5	110	9.984	0.001	0.0000	1000.0
6	120	0.000	0.000	0.0000	1000.0

Texture profile analysis

Texture profile analysis (TPA) of *shatadhautaghrita* and the nanolipogel was carried out using a CT3 texture analyser in TPA mode. TPA is a method used to determine mechanical properties in which a conical analytical probe (45°) is depressed twice into the sample at a test speed (2 mm/second in this study) to a depth (12 mm in the study). A predefined period is provided between the end of the first depression and the beginning of the second depression of *shatadhautaghrita* and the nanolipogel (Figure 4(a) and (b), respectively).

The maximum negative force on the graph indicates the adhesive force exerted by the sample; the more negative the value is, the more "sticky" it is. The area under the negative part of the graph is known as the adhesiveness (the energy required to break the probe–sample contact) and can give an indication of the cohesive forces between the molecules within the sample. The peak/maximum force is taken as a measure of the firmness; the higher the value is, the thicker the sample is.

Spreadability test

The spreadability of *shatadhautaghrita* and the nanolipogel were determined using the CT3 texture analyser in compression mode. Compression is a method of determining the spreadability pattern of a material. When a trigger force of 7 g has been developed, the conical analytical probe (45°) penetrates the sample at a test speed of 2 mm/second to a depth of 12 mm. During this time, the force required to penetrate the sample increases. When the specified penetration distance has been reached, the probe withdraws from the sample at the post-test speed of 2 mm/second. The maximum force value on the graph is a measure of the firmness of the sample at the specified depth. The area under the positive curve is a measure of the energy required to deform the sample to the defined distance (hardness work done). Research has shown that the firmness and energy required to deform a sample to a defined depth can be used to grade samples in order of spreadability. A higher peak load (firmness) and hardness work done value indicate a less spreadable sample. Conversely, a lower peak load (firmness) value coupled with a lower hardness work done value indicates a more spreadable sample. The spreadability values of *shatadhautaghrita* and the nanolipogel are shown in Figure 5(a) and (b), respectively.

Particle size

The average particle size of the *shatadhautaghrita* was evaluated using a Malvern zetasizer. The average particle size was found to be 388.2 nm with a PdIvalue of 0.536 shown in Figure 5(c). The average particle size of the optimized nanolipogel batch (F7) was found to be 359.4 nm, with a PdI value of 0.554 shown in Figure 5(d).

In-vitro drug release study

An *in-vitro* drug release study was conducted for plain fluconazole gel (without *shatadhautaghrita*), the fluconazole nanolipogel and the commercial formulation (0.5%). The release profile obtained is shown in Figure 6(a). It was observed that the release of the drug from the plain fluconazole gel, nanolipogel (F7) and commercial formulation was 29.36%, 80.50% and 72.24% shown in Table V.

Table V: *In-vitro* drug release study of plain gel, marketed formulation and nanolipogel (F7)

Time (min)	Plain Gel	Marketed Formulation (%)	F7 (%)
0	00	00	00
30	2.79	7.91	9.71
60	5.55	15.20	17.33
90	9.24	22.79	25.28
120	11.78	29.53	32.29
150	15.07	36.23	40.64
180	17.42	43.66	47.70
210	21.12	49.81	55.35
240	24.09	56.02	63.28
270	27.33	64.94	72.72
300	29.36	72.24	80.50

Release kinetics

The *in-vitro* release data were fitted to various release models, namely, the zero order, first order, matrix, Peppas and Hixson–Crowell models, and the best fit model was decided on the basis of the highest r^2 value. The Peppas model had the highest regression value (0.9943 for F7) and was found to be the best fit model for the nanolipogel formulations [Table VI near here].

Table VI: Release kinetics data of nanolipogel formulations (F7)

Zero order	First Order	Matrix	Peppas	Hixson–Crowell	Best fitting model
0.9869	0.9806	0.8799	0.9943	0.9829	Peppas

Ex-vivo drug permeation study

The results of the *ex-vivo* permeation study and the release profile obtained are shown in Figure 6(b). The release values of the drug from plain fluconazole gel, nanolipogel (F7) and commercial formulation were found to be 31.08%, 83.65% and 71.41%.[Table VII near here]

Table VII:*Ex-vivo* drug permeation study of plain gel, marketed formulation and nanolipogel (F7)

Time (min)	Plain Gel	Marketed Formulation (%)	F7 (%)
0	00	00	00
30	3.55	8.11	10.41
60	5.78	15.25	18.1
90	8.21	23.95	27.08
120	12.82	30.3	34.78
150	15.02	38.83	42.57
180	17.78	45.66	50.7
210	22.16	52.81	59.33
240	25.33	58.02	67.47
270	27.33	64.09	74.52
300	31.08	71.41	83.65

Release kinetics

The *ex-vivo* permeation data were fitted to various release models, namely, the zero order, first order, matrix, Peppas and Hixson–Crowell models, and the best fit model was decided on the basis of the highest r^2 value. The Peppas model had the highest regression value (0.9969 for F7) and was found to be the best fit model [Table VIII near here].

Table VIII: Release kinetics data of nanolipogel formulations (F7)

Zero order	First Order	Matrix	Peppas	Hixson–Crowell	Best fitting model
0.9879	0.9802	0.8803	0.9969	0.9853	Peppas

Antifungal activity study

In the antifungal studies the fungus used was *Candida albicans*. The zones of inhibition of F7 (18 mm) and the commercial formulation (16 mm) respectively. As shown in figure 7 (a) and (b).

Discussion

In this present research work the efforts were made to prepare nanolipogel using carbopol 934P, propylene glycol, methyl paraben, propyl paraben, TEA and *shatadhautaghrita*(SDG) as a penetration enhancer. The optimized formulation F7 of nanolipogel was white, smooth, viscous appearance having good texture, spredability and with particle size of 359.4 nm. Considering *in vitro* drug release of nanolipogel, has shown maximum release of drug (80.50%) as compare to plain fluconazole (without SDG) and commercial formulation(0.5%). The aim of incorporating *shatadhautaghrita*(SDG) as a penetration enhancer has successfully increased the penetration upto 83.65% examined via *Ex-vivo* permeation study. The Antifungal activity with zone of inhibition of F7 batch was 17mm, greater than commercial preparation(16mm).

Conclusions

The purpose of the present study was to develop a nanolipogel formulation of fluconazole using *shatadhautaghrita* for antifungal drug delivery. The present study showed that *shatadhautaghrita* may be used as a permeation enhancer in a topical drug delivery system for a poorly permeable drug like fluconazole to increase the permeation rate. The optimized batch showed higher drug release and antifungal activity compared with the commercial formulation. From the present study it can be concluded that the use of a nanolipogel is a better approach for increasing the release, permeation rate and antifungal activity of topical applications.

Acknowledgments

The authors thanks to Cipla Pharmaceuticals Ltd, Mumbai for providing fluconazole as gift samples for this work. We would also like to thanks Sanjivani College of Pharmaceutical Education and Research, Kopargaon, Maharashtra-423603, India. for providing required facilities to carry out this research work.

References

1. Agarwal S.: *Physical Pharmacy*, 2nd edn. CBS Publi&Distri PVT LTD India, 2012.

2. Basha N et al. Formulation and evaluation of gel containing fluconazole-antifungal agent, **Int J Drug Deve& Res.**, 2011, 3(4) 109-28.

3. Deshpande D et al. Shata-dhauta-ghrita- a case study. **INDIAN J TRADIT KNOW.**, 2009, 8(3) 387-391.

4. Dineshmohan D., Gupta V.: Transdermal delivery of fluconazole microsponges: Preparation and in vitro characterization. **J Drug Deli &Therp.**, 2016, 6(6) 7-15.

5. Helal D et al. Formulation and evaluation of fluconazole topical gel, **Int J Pharm Sci.**, 2012, 4(5) 176-183.

6. Jones DS et al. Examination of the flow rheological and textural properties of polymer gels composed of poly (methylvinylether-co-maleic anhydride) and poly (vinylpyrrolidone): Rheological and mathematical interpretation of textural parameters. **J Pharm Sci.**, 2002, 91(9) 2090-2101.

7. Kokare CK. *Pharmaceutical Microbiology: Experiment and Techniques*, 1st edn. Career Publications., 2005.

8. Kumar J et al. Anti-fungal activity of microemulsion based fluconazole gel for onychomycosis against aspergillusniger, **Int J Pharm Pharm Sci.**, 2012, 5(1) 96-102.

9. Osmani RA et al. Novel cream containing microsponges of anti acne agent: formulation development and evaluation, **Cur Drug Del.**, 2015, (12) 504-416.

10. Pande V et al. Design expert assisted formulation of topical bioadhesive gel of sertaconazole nitrate, **Adv Pharm Bull.**, 2014, 4(2) 121-130.

11. Patel R et al. Formulation and evaluation of carbopol gel containing liposomes of ketoconazole., (Part-II). **Int. J. Drug Deliv. Technol.**, 2009, 1(2) 42-45.

12. Phadtare G et al. Formulation and evaluation of topical antifungal gel containing fluconazole., **Eur J Pharm Med Res**., 2016, 3(7) 365-368.

13. Sharma PP. *Cosmetic's Formulation Manufacturing Quality Control*, 5[th]edn. Vandana Publication, 2014.

14. Swetha C et al. Formulation and evaluation of clarithromycin topical gel., **Int J Drug Dev& Res.**, 2013, 5(4) 194-202.

15. VermaA et al.Formulation, optimization and evaluation of clobetasol propionate gel.,**Int J of Pharm Sci.**, 2013, 5(4) 666-674.

16. http://www.brookfieldengineering.com/education/applications/texture-moisturizing-cream-spreadability.asp.

18. Bidwai, V. R., Gumble, S. P., Pawade, S., Deshmukh, A. R., & Morey, M.: Shatdhauta Ghrita - A Evaluation Study in Pediatrics. *Pediatrics & Health Research.*, 2018, *03*(01), 2–4.

19. Dhauta, S., Case, G. A., Deshpande, S., Deshpande, A., Tupkari, S., & Agnihotri, A. (2014). Shata- dhauta- ghrita – A case study, (May 2009).

YOUR KNOWLEDGE HAS VALUE

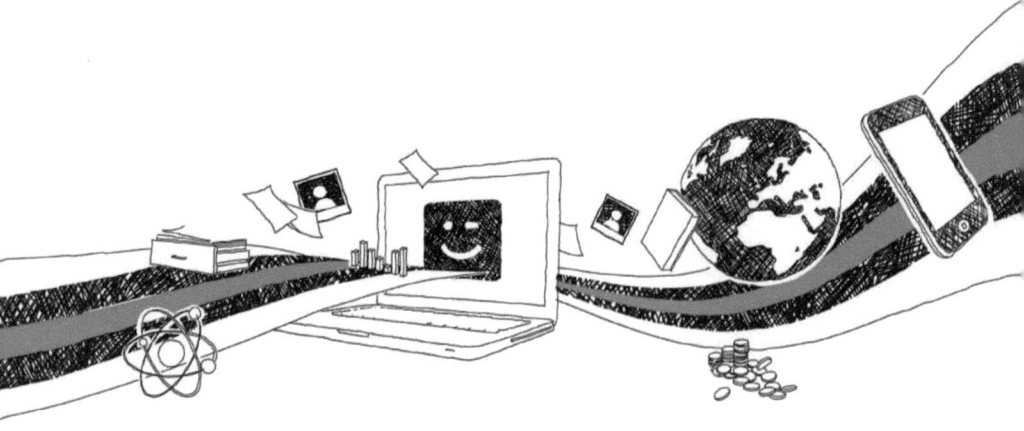

- - We will publish your bachelor's and
    master's thesis, essays and papers

- - Your own eBook and book -
    sold worldwide in all relevant shops

- - Earn money with each sale

Upload your text at www.GRIN.com
and publish for free

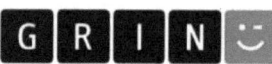